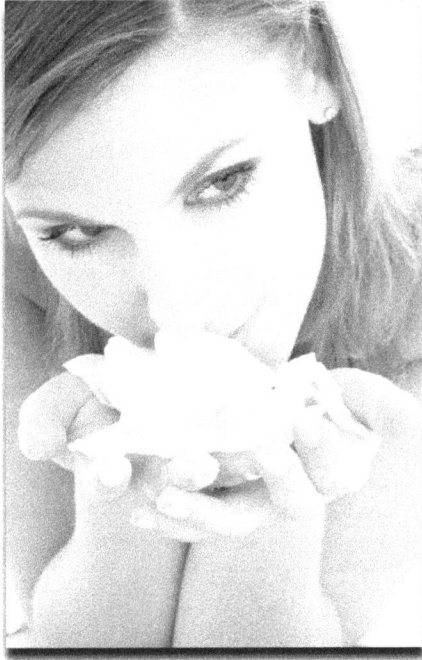

A DIY Guide to Therapeutic Bath Enhancements

Homemade Recipes for
Bath Salts, Melts, Bombs and Scrubs
(The Art of the Bath Vol. 2)

Alynda Carroll

Ordinary Matters Publishing
P.O. Box 430577
Houston, TX 77243

www.OrdinaryMattersPublishing.com

A DIY Guide to Therapeutic Bath Enhancements
Homemade Recipes for Bath Salts, Melts, Bombs and Scrubs

ISBN-13: 978-1-941303-09-2 (paperback)
ISBN-10: 1941303099
First Printing: October, 2014

Printed in the United States of America

Books by Alynda Carroll

The Art of the Bath Series

Custom Massage Therapy Oils
A DIY Guide to Therapeutic Recipes for Homemade Massage Oils

A DIY Guide to Therapeutic Bath Enhancements
Homemade Recipes for Bath Salts, Melts, Bombs & Scrubs

A DIY Guide to Therapeutic Body & Skin Care Recipes
Homemade Body Lotions, Skin Creams, Gels, Whipped Butters,
Herbal Balms and Salves

A DIY Guide to Therapeutic Spa Treatments
Homemade Recipes for the Face, Hands, Feet & Body

A DIY Guide to Therapeutic Body Butters
A Beginner's Guide to Homemade Body and Hair Butters

A DIY Guide to Therapeutic Natural Hair Care Recipes
A Beginner's Guide to Homemade Shampoos, Conditioners,
Rinses, Gels and Sprays

Life Hacks for Everyday Living Series

HOUSEHOLD HACKS
Super Simple Ways to Clean Your Home Effortlessly Using
Hydrogen Peroxide and Other Cleaning Secrets

Pick up your FREE report *Learn the Art of Self-Massage*:

http://www.ordinarymatterspublishing.com/massage-bonus

Praise for *The Art of the Bath* series

for *A DIY Guide to Therapeutic Spa Treatments from the Comfort of Your Home*

"Ahhhh this is a keeper! It's packed with awesome and easy to make spa like treatments. I love going to the spa, but in between spa treatments this book is as good as it gets. My favorites so far are the healthy coconut cuticle softener, the tension-relieving eucalyptus food massage oil treatment- so good oh and for a coffee junkie like me, the all-over coffee body scrub priceless! Great DIY spa treatments book."
~ Yvette (Amazon reviewer)

for *A DIY Guide to Therapeutic Bath Enhancements*

". . . easy to follow and very simple too. If you are looking for an book that you can easily follow and make you feel like a pro in no time when it comes to making soaps, bath salts and scrubs, this is the book to have!"
~ LH Thompson (Amazon reviewer)

for *Custom Massage Therapy Oils*

As well as being relaxing, the benefits of massage can be physical as well as mental. This book is a great little guide to their therapeutic benefits, how to make your own massage oil and which blends are recommended to induce sleep, invigorate or enliven, boost the immune system and more. I will be taking the advice in this book on board, as I know how wonderful massage oils can be - it's just a case of knowing which ones are right to use, depending on the mood and/ or benefits you want to induce in the person receiving the massage." ~ Anna J (Amazon reviewer)

for *The Art of the Bath series*

"I love Carroll's DIY Bath series. They are all so welcoming and are full of all these great ideas. Must have." ~ Laura Pope (Amazon reviewer)

"Everything is a miracle. It is a miracle that one does not dissolve in one's bath like a lump of sugar."

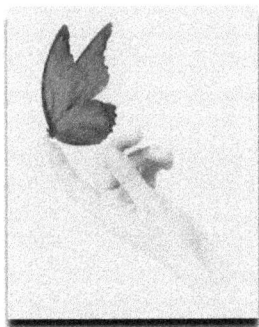

~ Pablo Picasso

A Note to the Reader

Are you a bath or a shower person? It seems like we're either one or the other, doesn't it? I've been a life-long bath lover. There is something wonderful and luxurious about sinking into a tub of hot water and allowing the water to rise around you. I love it. So it shouldn't be a big surprise if I tell you how much I've enjoyed traveling the road to perfect the Art of the Bath—and art it is.

A true bath is way more than a means to get clean. It's a sensual full-body experience. When I was young, it was all about relaxation, warmth, and luxury. Today, many years later, the bath is all that and more. Now it's still about relaxation, but I'm also focused on ways to alleviate pain, combat insomnia, and much more. Imagine my delight when I discovered the modern world of aromatherapy. Now I want to share it all with you.

ALYNDA CARROLL

x

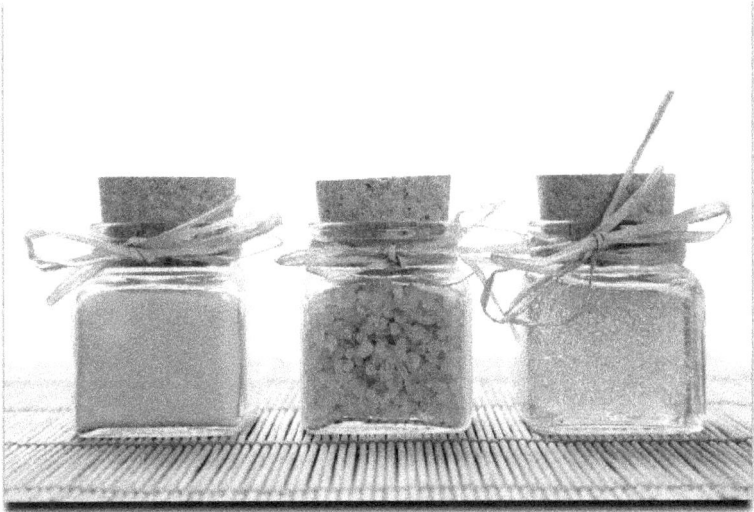

How to Give Yourself A Massage

Thank you for buying this book. In appreciation, I'm offering you this free report:

Learn the Art of Self-Massage

http://www.ordinarymatterspublishing.com/massage-bonus/

CONTENTS

INTRODUCTION

"There must be quite a few things a hot bath won't cure, but I don't know many of them ." —Sylvia Plath, *The Bell Jar*

The History of the Bath

For centuries, immersing oneself and soaking in water has been part of the world's culture. Taking baths began as part of religious rituals and as a means of socializing, and is still used in this way today. Bathing for personal hygiene started to increase in the 18th century, when the correlation between cleanliness and good health began to be believed. Since then, the use of hydrotherapy has become widespread in helping in the rehabilitation and healing of bodily injuries. One of the most widely held uses for bathing today is the relaxation and the restorative qualities it provides.

The popularity of bathing as a meditative and restorative experience has encouraged those who practice aromatherapy to create ways of combining the two. To infuse the bathwater with fragrances that will aid or enhance mind, body, and spiritual healing, many products have been developed, including bath salts, scrubs, melts, and bath bombs. These easy-to-make products can take a normal bathroom and create a spa-like experience, even for someone who has never set foot in a spa.

Aromatherapy

I would imagine that if you have had a massage, you've encountered aromatherapy. You may not have known it, but you probably did. Massage therapists have embraced aromatherapy and all its benefits.

What is Aromatherapy?

Some people think aromatherapy is simply the use of essential oils consisting of plant compounds that give off a good smell, and the use of the oils to create a better environment through the sense of smell. They relate it to the oils placed on the hot lamps so that the scent is activated and fills the room. To the extent that the sense of smell and essential oils are used, that is true. However, aromatherapy is much more than that.

Today aromatherapy is numbered among the many rising alternative medicine therapies that are gaining more and more acceptance. It involves the use of essential oils and other plant compounds to heal the body and the mind. In some places, aromatherapy also has a spiritual component.

We all know that studies have shown the power of smell in relationship to memory. So it shouldn't be too much of a leap to realize that the power of scent can help us in even more ways. Sure, it makes us feel good, but the benefit doesn't stop there. Aromatherapy has developed into therapy that affords great healing to the mind and the body. More and more studies are confirming the benefits of these various plant essential oils, and more and more people are finding that their bodies are responding to the various treatments.

Aromatherapy and the Bath

Okay, so aromatherapy can probably be traced back to the days of good old Cleopatra when she dipped her toe into the ancient Egyptian bath. I'm sure she knew the value of a good restorative bath as well as anyone and she was no stranger to perfumed oils. The Egyptians used aromatherapy for massages, in religious ceremonies, and even in their famous embalming process, but the use of scented oils actually dates back to the Stone Age. Aromatherapy has been a world-wide experience around the world for thousands of years.

Today the benefits of aromatherapy continue to grow as more and more studies are performed, confirm the benefits traditionally held, and discover even more. There are definite proven benefits emotionally and physically associated with aromatherapy.

Who hasn't yearned for a hot bath when their body is worn and torn? Who doesn't remember the calming effect of hot water beating down on their tight muscles when their backs are in spasm? Think about the medicinal properties of Epson salts. Now, add the benefits of essential oils and you're on your way to a more enhanced bathing experience with definite therapeutic benefits.

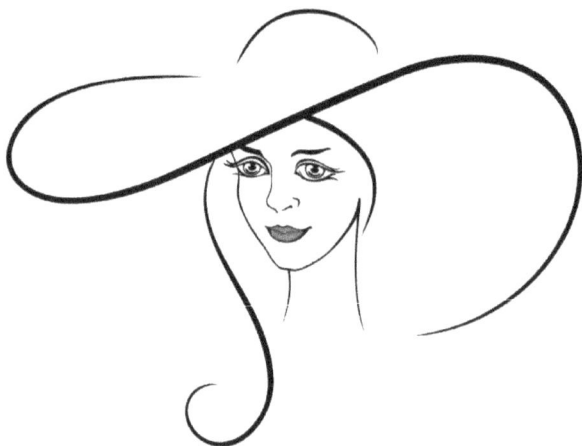

Bath Enhancements

What they Are and What they Do

Bath products have come a long way in the last few decades. At one time, there weren't many ways to truly explore the art of the bath. I remember making herbal sachets and attaching them to the tub faucet so they would hang, and the water would fall onto them and release the herbal scents. Not today. It's way more sophisticated. We're only going to focus on the four main modern bath products that most people enjoy and can easily make. You may not be familiar with the various terms being used such as bath salts, bombs, melts, and scrubs, but you're going to love the results.

Bath Salts

Most bath salts contain Epsom salts (magnesium chloride) and sea salt (sodium chloride), which can change the osmotic balance of water. This change is beneficial to the bather, helping soften the water and, with the addition of natural vegetable oils, helps alleviate dry skin, as well as gently exfoliate calluses.

Bath Bombs

Bath bombs contain bath salts, so they provide the same restorative qualities, and they also contain sodium bicarbonate or baking soda, which aids in cleansing the skin. The additions of citric acid in bath bombs make them fizz when immersed in water, adding an unexpected tactile sensation to the experience.

Bath Melts
The rich and creamy addition of butters, such as cocoa and Shea, make bath melts especially effective for those with dry skin. These bath aids slowly dissolve, for a subtle infusion of added nutrient-rich oils.

Bath Scrubs
Bath scrubs are used for exfoliating. By using natural salts and sugars, the body gets a gentle scrub that effectively gets rid of dead skin cells, and leave skin feeling smooth and rejuvenated. The circular motion used to apply bath scrubs also increases circulation.

To Melt or to Bomb
Bath melts have only recently been added to the bather's mood-enhancing selections. They're subtle. They're slower than the sudden action of a bath bomb when it hits the bath water. Instead of the heady fizzing of a bomb, a melt does exactly what its name says: it dissolves slowly into the warm bath water. You may have heard the melts called "tub truffles" or "tub treats." They are two different bath items comprised of different ingredients. In a hurry? Go with the bath bomb. Ready to soak and take it easy? A melt is your best choice

Benefits of Essential Oils

There are many kinds of essential oils, way more than we will address here. To make this a little easier for you, only the oils listed in the recipes will be provided here under their therapeutic benefit.

Anxiety
Chamomile (Roman), Geranium, Lavender, Jasmine, Orange, Sandalwood

Antidepressant
Lavender, Orange

Anti-rheumatic
Blue Violet Leaf, Chamomile, Cedarwood, Lemon, Lavender

Arthritis
Blue Violet Leaf

Concentration (lack of) | Focus (lack of)
Ginger, Sandalwood

Energy (lack of)
Lemon, Orange

Fatigue
Rose

Headache | Migraine
Lavender, Blue Violet Leaf, Chamomile (Roman)

Insomnia
Chamomile (Roman), Lavender, Sandalwood

Irritability
Geranium, Lavender, Sandalwood

Memory loss
Rosemary

Muscle pains
Chamomile (Roman),

Overwork, Overwhelmed
Lavender

Relaxation (lack of)
Geranium, Jasmine, Lavender, Sandalwood

Rheumatism
Cedarwood, Chamomile (German), Lavender, Lemon

Sedative
Cedarwood, Jasmine, Lavender, Rose, Sandalwood

Shock
Lavender

Skin
Sunflower, Cedarwood

Sunburn | Windburn
Chamomile (Roman), Lavender

Depression
Jasmine

Restlessness
Lemon, Lemon Verbena, Geranium

ESSENTIAL OILS USED IN RECIPES

Apricot Kernel

Chamomile (German)

Chamomile (Roman)

Eucalyptus

Geranium

Lavender

Lemon

Jasmine

Orange

Patchouli

Rose

Sandalwood

Sunflower

Sweet Almond

Violet Leaf

Blue Violet Leaf

Wintergreen

Getting Started

It's easy to make bath products right in your own kitchen. In fact, most of the ingredients are ones you probably already have on hand.

Common Ingredients
Common ingredients for making bath salts, scrubs, bombs, and melts include:

Salts – Preferably Epsom salts and sea salts

Oils – Vegetable oils are best, and may include Apricot Kernel oil, Sweet Almond oil, olive oil, Jojoba oil, sunflower oil, and grape seed oil. Mineral oil can be substituted.

Sugar – Plain, white table sugar is the easiest and most available to use, although a more coarse salt choice can provide further exfoliation.

Essential oils – The range of essential oils is broad, and limited only by your personal preference and/or skin sensitivity. It is advisable to test a drop on the skin before using, to eliminate the possibility of a reaction.

Coloring – Food coloring may be used, but it is best to dilute it before adding since it can stain the skin. Soap colorants are skin-safe and will not stain.

Dried flowers, petals and herbs – These add texture and a note of luxury to the bath.

For making melts, some of the ingredients listed above are used. In addition to those, the most important ingredient in bath melts is the butter. Cocoa butter is easy to melt and has pleasing effects, but Shea butter has more emollient properties, making it the preferred choice.

SAFETY FIRST!

If there is any doubt about how you will react to any of the ingredients in the making of bath products, it is wise to test a small amount on your skin before making the bath. Although these products are made of natural ingredients, you should never ingest them. Essential oils are the volatile aroma compounds from plants, and are potentially hazardous. They can cause irritation, allergic reaction, and/or become toxic with extended use. It is recommended that pregnant woman and children NOT be exposed to essential oils. Also, since salts have a drying effect, if you suffer from dry skin, you should use those products which include salt with caution.

If there is any doubt about how you will react to any of the ingredients in these recipes, it is wise to test a small amount on your skin before using. Also, although these products are made of natural ingredients, you should never ingest them.

Wintergreen
Wintergreen has a reputation for helping with arthritis and many other health problems, but caution is needed.

Wintergreen has analgesic properties, and should therefore not be taken by anyone who has problems with aspirin or aspirin-like products. It is also suggested that anyone who is taking blood-thinning medications not use Wintergreen.

You should definitely read up on these and other oils to make sure you know whether it is appropriate oil for you and your needs.

Basic Directions

General directions for bath bombs when mixing dry and wet ingredients

To mix the dry and wet ingredients together, pour the wet mixture into a squirt bottle, and squirt the liquid onto the dry ingredient mix to reduce activating the fizzing of the citric acid. After the liquid mixture has been added to the dry ingredients, whisk the entire mixture together.

The right ratio of wet to dry will be achieved when a handful of the mixture keeps it shaped when squeezed, without crumbling. If crumbling occurs, spritz the mixture with another teaspoon of distilled water or until desired density is achieved.

How to Mold Bath Melts

Pour mixture into molds, and place in the refrigerator until completely hardened, approximately one hour. Carefully remove from molds, being careful not to handle too long, since the heat of the skin can begin the melting process.

Wrap in foil or cellophane, or place in decorative vase or jar.

Add one melt to a warm bath and enjoy!

How to Use Bath Scrubs

To use, apply a small handful to wet skin and gently scrub with your hand or a washcloth in a circular motion. Rinse well and pat skin dry. (Not for use on the face.)

Store in an airtight container.

Presentation and Storage

Bath salts, scrubs, bath bombs, and melts make wonderful gifts for birthdays, baby or wedding showers, holidays, or any special days. These are gifts easy enough for children to make. You can get as creative as you want when it comes to how to package and present them. Use molds, containers, and wrapping choices found at your local craft or department store.

How to Use Bath Melts and Bombs

The bath bomb mixture can be molded into many shapes, either by hand or using molds such as plastic Easter eggs, candy/soap molds, or specially made bath bomb molds. If using a two-part mold, such as a plastic egg, pack the mixture firmly into each side of the egg and then join the two molds together. Gently release the newly formed bath bomb from the mold, and place on a clean surface. Allow to dry for several hours before packaging or using.

What to Use to Make Bath Melts or Bombs

To mold your melts and bombs, the sky's the limit as to the size and shape you can achieve. Go where your imagination takes you, using:

- Mini Muffin Tins

- Plastic Easter Eggs

o   Clear Plastic Christmas Tree Ornaments

o   Ice Cube Trays

o   Candy Molds

o   Cake Molds

o   Soap Molds

o   Butter Molds

Containers to Use for Bath Salts

Containers for salts and scrubs should be airtight. For added convenience, include a small scoop to make it easy to add under the running water in the bath. You can find unusual containers at thrift shops, yard sales, and specialty shops. Oh, and don't throw out that sauce, jam, or condiment jar after you're finished. By removing the labels and washing and drying thoroughly, you have an instant container waiting to be filled. A little hint for gift giving; use cellophane envelopes, foil wrap, or fabric drawstring pouches. These are easily made or can also be purchased at your local craft store.

Bath Salt Recipes

REXLAXING APRICOT-LAVENDER BATH SALTS

Nothing is more relaxing than a lavender-scented bath. Lavender is a popular herb known for its many beneficial properties. Its scent alone calms the nerves and relieves tension. Those who suffer from insomnia, anxiety, and even nervous stomachs have been known to sing this herb's praises. Today herbalists often tout lavender to those who suffer migraines in menopause.

For our purposes, lavender salts are great antidotes for stress and anxiety, but also help with aches, muscle, and joint stiffness, pain, and rheumatic discomfort. A good lavender soak is a great prelude to relaxing sleep.

In this recipe, Apricot Kernel oil is added for its anti-inflammatory properties as well as its soothing pain-relieving qualities.

Ingredients:
2 cups Epsom salts
2 tsps. Apricot Kernel oil
8 drops Lavender essential oil*

Directions:

Put Epsom salts into large bowl. Add the Apricot Kernel oil a little at a time, while stirring to mix thoroughly. Add the Lavender essential oil drop by drop until thoroughly combined. (Use more or less essential oil until it is the scent strength you prefer.)

Add ¼ cup of bath salt, under running water, to the bath and enjoy!

Store in airtight container for up to three months.

Be sure and use half the suggested dose of lavender oil if you are elderly, disabled, or are preparing a bath or shower for a young child.

Alternative

Not in the mood for a bath? Take a lavender shower. Add three drops of lavender oil to one capful of water and pour onto your wet hair. Stay under the shower as the lavender oil rinses off your head and body. Feel free to catch the lavender water in your cupped hands and breathe in the relaxing scent. Be sure and add a few drops of lavender oil to your shampoo. Rinse as usual.

SOOTHING ROSE-GERANIUM BATH SALTS

Both rose and geranium are relaxing floral scents that are soothing and reminiscent of being in a garden. That alone is enough to produce some relaxation, but if you really want to pamper yourself, add dry rose petals.

Massage therapists love Sweet Almond oil for its sweet, soothing fragrance and its ability to relieve stiff and sore muscles. The oil is also terrific for dry skin. Recent studies have demonstrated that Rose oil is a definite help with anxiety and stress. Apparently Rose oil not only helps with feelings of relaxation and calm, but also may help lower a person's breathing rate. Studies have also noted the oil's mood-boosting properties and its ability to help with depression and headache. Geranium oil has anti-inflammatory, antidepressant, and sedative properties. It is often used to combat insomnia, nervousness, and even anger.

The combination of these three oils produces a salt that is well worth trying if you are feeling overwhelmed, stressed, or feeling full of aches and pains.

Ingredients:
2 cups Epsom salts
2 tsps. Sweet Almond oil*
4 drops Rose essential oil
2 drops Geranium essential oil

Directions:

Put Epsom salts in a large bowl. Slowly add Sweet Almond oil, while stirring constantly to mix well. Add Rose essential oil, and then Geranium essential oil, drop by drop, while continuing to stir. (You can adjust the amount of essential oils to your desired scent strength but remember their sedative effects.)

Add ¼ cup of bath salt under running water to the bath and enjoy!

Store in a decorative, airtight container, for up to three months.

Alternative

For a more citrus flavor, substitute the ever-popular Sweet Orange oil. Definitely a stress-reducer. Add 6 - 8 drops.

JASMINE BATH SALTS

The sweet floral scent of jasmine evokes romance and calming thoughts. Sea salts soften the water, while Epsom salts add muscle relaxing minerals.

Sunflower oil is great for those with sensitive skin. It has a light texture and a light scent, so it won't compete with the scents of other oils. This is a great oil to soften the skin. You'll love this oil if you suffer from dry skin or eczema. The best way to achieve the full benefits of sunflower oil on the skin is to make sure you use it in or after a hot shower or bath, so as a component in bath salts, it does a great job. The warmth of the bath will help the oil soak into your skin.

Jasmine is an oil with a distinctive scent and great benefits. I love the scent of jasmine and have Jasmine plants placed around my back yard so the scent greets me where ever I go. It offers instant relaxation. Jasmine also lifts my mood. Great oil for relaxation, but also an aid for those who are caught in the midst of negativity or feeling down in the dumps.

Ingredients:
1 cup Epsom salts
1 cup Sea salt
2 tsps. Sunflower oil
6 drops Jasmine essential oil*

Directions

Mix salts together in a large bowl. Slowly add the sunflower oil, while stirring constantly to mix well. Add Jasmine essential oil, drop by drop, while stirring, until desired scent strength is achieved.

Use ¼ cup of bath salt, adding under running water to dissolve into the bath and enjoy!

Store in an airtight container for up to three months.

Alternative

Maybe you don't want to get too relaxed. You'd prefer bath salts with a bit of a kick. If that's the case, try Patchouli oil. Benefits include its ability to fight lethargy.

LEMON-CHAMOMILE GOOD MOOD BATH SALTS

Who doesn't respond to the scent of lemon? Lemon is refreshing and conjures cheerful thoughts and feelings. Chamomile is the scent of comfort. Combine the two, and you have a bath experience that's sure to put you in a good mood.

Apricot Kernel oil brings its pain-relieving anti-inflammatory properties to this bath salt recipe. Lemon oil is known for its ability to combat mental fatigue, anxiety, exhaustion, and nervousness. It is refreshing and makes you suddenly feel alert. Oddly, some people say lemon oil helps them fight insomnia. Chamomile oil is probably most associated with its calming effect, but there are many more reasons why chamomile is a good addition to this recipe. It's known to lift depression and cause a change in mood for the better. The anti-inflammatory and pain-relieving properties are a huge benefit, too.

Ingredients:
1 cup Epsom salts
1 cup Sea salt
2 tsps. Apricot Kernel oil
2 drops Lemon essential oil
3 drops Chamomile essential oil*

Directions:

Mix salts together in a large bowl. Slowly add the Apricot Kernel oil, while stirring constantly, to mix well. Add Lemon and Chamomile essential oils, drop by drop, while stirring, until desired scent strength is achieved.

Use ¼ cup of bath salt, adding under running water to dissolve into the bath and enjoy!

Store in an airtight container for up to three months.

Alternative

There are two types of chamomile oil, the Roman and the German. The Roman Chamomile oil is used more for its calming effects. This smells a bit like apples and is more commonly used for aromatherapy. The German or Blue Chamomile oil has stronger anti-inflammatory properties and is considered good for those suffering from arthritis and rheumatism. It has a deeper blue color. The German seems to be the more popular of the two except in Britain. Depending on your needs, you may want to try both.

Chamomile is a member of the ragweed family, so test the oil first if you suffer from a ragweed allergy.

CEDARWOOD BATH SALTS

The woody fragrance of Cedar wood evokes warm feelings of being by a comforting fire on a cold wintry day. Combined with the healing properties of Epsom salts, this bath is both stress-reducing and strengthening.

Recent tests point to Cedarwood oil's positive effects for those suffering from arthritis and joint and tissue inflammation. The oil's anti-inflammatory properties can ease the pain and discomfort of sufferers. In addition, Cedarwood oil is a strong sedative. It is good for the mind as well as for the body. It relieves inflammation and is great for itchy skin. Insomnia sufferers turn to Cedarwood for its benefit of calm, restorative sleep. The oil also benefits those who suffer from stress, depression, and chronic anxiety.

The addition of the Sweet Almond oil adds a dimension of fragrance as well as the benefit of softening the skin.

Ingredients:
2 cups Epsom salts
2 tsps. Sweet Almond oil
3 drops Cedarwood essential oil*

Directions:

Mix salts together in a large bowl. Slowly add the Sweet Almond oil, while stirring constantly to mix well. Add the Cedarwood essential oil, drop by drop, while stirring, until desired scent strength is achieved.

Use ¼ cup of bath salt, adding under running water to dissolve into the bath and enjoy!

Store in an airtight container for up to three months.

Alternative

Cedarwood oil is often used in place of Sandalwood oil. Sandalwood, a more expensive oil, has a strong scent and is known for its ability to trigger deep relaxation. Many use this oil for deep meditation. Other benefits include concentration and calmness.

If you have sensitive skin, test the Cedarwood oil. In high concentrations, skin irritation could occur. A little bit goes a long way.

Bath Bomb Recipes

LIVE-IT-UP EUCALYPTUS BATH BOMB

The scent of eucalyptus works as a decongestant when inhaled, and is said to be invigorating and revitalizing.

Ingredients:
2 cups Baking soda
1 cup Powdered citric acid
1 cup Corn starch
1 cup Epsom salts
2 tbsps. distilled water
2 tsps. Eucalyptus essential oil
2-3 drops food coloring (optional)

Directions:
In a large bowl, sift together baking soda, powdered citric acid, corn starch, and Epsom salts. Stir to mix thoroughly. In a smaller bowl, pour in the distilled water and add the food coloring, stirring well until food coloring is thoroughly diluted. Next, add Eucalyptus essential oil, drop by drop, until desired scent strength is reached.

Mixing Directions:
Follow the general directions when mixing dry and wet ingredients.

Molding Bath Bombs
Go to how to mold bath melts and bombs.

LEMON-VERBENA BATH BOMB

The sweet floral fragrance of Verbena combines well with lemon for an uplifting and renewing bath experience.

Ingredients:
1 cup Epsom salts
2 cups Baking soda
1 cup Corn starch
1 cup powdered citric acid
2 tbsps. distilled water
1 tsp lemon essential oil
1 tsp Verbena essential oil
2-3 drops food coloring (optional)

Directions:
In a large bowl, sift together baking soda, powdered citric acid, corn starch and Epsom salts. Stir to mix thoroughly. In a smaller bowl pour in the distilled water, and add the food coloring, stirring well until food coloring is thoroughly diluted. Next, add lemon and verbena essential oils, drop by drop, until desired scent strength is reached.

Mixing Directions:
Follow the general directions when mixing dry and wet ingredients.

Molding Bath Bombs
Go to how to mold bath melts and bombs.

VIOLET BATH BOMB

The old-fashioned fragrance of violets conjures the charm of a bygone Victorian era of proper manners and sweet nosegays. The use of violet leaf oil goes back to the time of Homer and Virgil, and is known for its calming, relaxing, soothing, and even inspiring attributes. (Recent tests confirm the effects of blue violet leaf oil on headaches and aches and pains.)

Ingredients:
1 cup Epsom salts
2 cups Baking soda
1 cup Corn starch
1 cup Powdered citric acid
2 tbsps. Distilled water
2 tsps. Violet Leaf essential oil
Dried violet or pansy petals (optional)
2-3 drops food coloring (optional)

Directions:
In a large bowl, sift together baking soda, powdered citric acid, corn starch and Epsom salts. Add violet or pansy petals. Stir to mix thoroughly. In a smaller bowl, pour in the distilled water and add the food coloring, stirring well until food coloring is thoroughly diluted. Next, add violet essential oil, drop by drop, until desired scent strength is reached.

Mixing Directions:
Follow the general directions when mixing dry and wet ingredients.

Molding Bath Bombs

Go to how to mold bath melts and bombs.

ORANGE BLOSSOM BATH BOMB

The sweet citrus scent of orange is refreshing and restorative. It is the scent of comfort and hope. If you're looking for something to pick up your mood and soothe your anxiety, gives this a try.

Ingredients:
1 cup Epsom salts
2 cups Baking soda
1 cup Corn starch
1 cup powdered citric acid
2 tbsps. distilled water
2 tsps. Orange essential oil
2-3 drops food coloring (optional)

Directions:
In a large bowl, sift together baking soda, powdered citric acid, corn starch and Epsom salts. Stir to mix thoroughly. In a smaller bowl pour in the distilled water and add the food coloring, stirring well until food coloring is thoroughly diluted. Next, add orange essential oil, drop by drop, until desired scent strength is reached.

Mixing Directions:
Follow the general directions when mixing dry and wet ingredients.

Molding Bath Bombs
Go to how to mold bath melts and bombs.

WHITE-GERANIUM BATH BOMB

These beautiful white bath bombs look luxurious in any bathroom and offer a subtle tropical floral scent that is both soothing and purifying. Geranium is known for its calming and revitalizing effects. Want to reduce stress and frustration, give this recipe a try.

Ingredients:
1 cup Epsom salts
2 cups Baking soda
1 cup Corn starch
1 cup Powdered citric acid
2 tbsps. Distilled water
2 tsps. White Geranium essential oil

Directions:
In a large bowl, sift together baking soda, powdered citric acid, corn starch and Epsom salts. Stir to mix thoroughly. In a smaller bowl pour in the distilled water and add the food coloring, stirring well until food coloring is thoroughly diluted. Next, add essential oil, drop by drop, until desired scent strength is reached.

Mixing Directions:
Follow the general directions when mixing dry and wet ingredients.

Molding Bath Bombs
Go to the section on how to mold bath melts and bombs

Bath Melt Recipes

PATCHOULI BATH MELT

The scent of patchouli oil has an earthy, muskiness that is at the same time both soothing and stimulating.

Ingredients:
1 cup Cocoa butter
½ cup Grape seed oil
10 drops Patchouli essential oil
Soap colorant (optional)

Directions:

In a large microwave-safe measuring cup or bowl, or in a double boiler on top of the stove, melt the cocoa butter. Add Grape seed oil and mix thoroughly. Add, drop by drop, the patchouli essential oil, until desired scent strength is achieved. Colorant may also be added. Mix well.

To Mold

Go to general directions how to mold melts.

LEMON TEA TREE BATH MELT

Tea tree oil has antiseptic properties, making this bath melt a healing aid as well as a soothing bath additive.

Ingredients:
1 cup Shea butter
½ cup Olive Oil
6 drops Tea Tree essential oil
3 drops lemon essential oil
Soap colorant (optional)

Directions:

Use a double boiler on top of the store or a rather large microwave-safe measuring cup or bowl, and melt the Shea butter. Add olive oil and mix thoroughly. Add, drop by drop, the tea tree and lemon essential oils, until desired scent strength is achieved. Colorant may also be added. Mix well.

To Mold

Go to general directions how to mold melts.

ROSE BATH MELT

For a romantic bath, there's nothing like the scent of roses to conjure the happiness of receiving big bouquets or ambling through beautiful gardens. It's also said that there's nothing quite like rose oil to fight depression, stress, and fatigue.

Ingredients:
1 cup Shea butter
½ cup Apricot Kernel oil
10 drops Rose essential oil
Dried rose petals
Soap colorant (optional)

Directions:

In a large microwave-safe measuring cup or bowl, or in a double boiler on top of the stove, melt the Shea butter. Add apricot kernel oil and mix thoroughly. Add, drop by drop, the rose essential oil, until desired scent strength is achieved. Colorant may also be added. Mix well.

To Mold

Before pouring mixture into molds, place a pinch of dried rose petals into the bottom of the mold.

Go to general directions how to mold melts.

GLITTERING FRANKINCENSE AND MYRRH BATH MELT

Frankincense and Myrrh are the oils valued for their abilities to help you become more focused and centered. Both have a warm, musky scent for a relaxing bath experience.

Ingredients:
1 cup Cocoa butter
½ cup Sweet Almond oil
5 drops Frankincense essential oil
5 drops Myrrh essential oil
Gold glitter (optional)
Soap colorant (optional)

Directions:

Choose a large microwave-safe measuring cup or bowl. (You can also use a double boiler on top of the stove.) Melt the cocoa butter. Add sweet almond oil and mix thoroughly. Add, drop by drop, the frankincense and myrrh essential oils, until desired scent strength is achieved. Colorant may also be added. Mix well.

To Mold

Here's a great option: Before pouring into molds, add a pinch of gold glitter in the bottom of the each mold.

Go to general directions how to mold melts.

PEPPERMINT BATH MELT

Peppermint oil has a crisp scent that has that wake-up effect on a person's senses. The mind is revived and the fatigue is gone. While this is a year-round recipe, it doesn't hurt to remember that this invigorating bath melt would make an excellent Christmas or holiday gift.

Ingredients:
1 cup Cocoa butter
½ cup Sweet Almond oil
5 -10 drops Peppermint essential oil*
Soap colorant (optional)

Directions:

In a large microwave-safe measuring cup or bowl, or in a double boiler on top of the stove, melt the cocoa butter. Add sweet almond oil and mix thoroughly. Add, drop by drop, the peppermint essential oil, until desired scent strength is achieved. Colorant may also be added. Mix well.

To Mold

Go to general directions how to mold melts.

Peppermint oil can be strong for some, so use cautiously at first as too much oil may burn sensitive skin.

Bath Scrub Recipes

None of the following bath scrub recipes are for the face.

ALMOND BATH SCRUB

Almonds provide the right balance of gentle abrasion when mixed with salt. Jojoba oil is ultra-moisturizing, making this the perfect scrub for dry skin.

Ingredients:
½ cup blanched almonds
½ cup Sea salt
½ cup Epsom salts
Jojoba oil to cover
1 drop Almond extract (optional)

Directions:
Place almonds in a food processor and pulse until coarsely ground. In a large bowl, combine ground almonds with sea salt and Epsom salts. Cover the mixture completely with jojoba oil and mix well. Add a drop of almond extract to the mixture and mix thoroughly.

Follow the general directions on how to use bath scrubs.

OATMEAL VANILLA BATH SCRUB

Oatmeal works to gently remove dry, dead skin and leaves it feeling smooth and rejuvenated.

Ingredients:
½ cup Oatmeal
½ cup Sea salt
½ cup Epsom salts
¼ cup Apricot Kernel oil
1 drop Vanilla extract

Directions:
In a food processer, add oatmeal and pulse until coarsely ground. Place ground oatmeal into a large bowl, and add sea salt and Epsom salts. Mix well. While continuing to stir, slowly add the Apricot kernel oil, until ingredients are well combined. Add a drop of vanilla extract and stir again.

Follow the general directions on how to use bath scrubs.

LAVENDER SUGAR BATH SCRUB

Using the white sugar and olive oil you already have in your pantry makes this bath scrub economical enough to make lavender-scented bath scrubs for everyone on your gift list.

Ingredients:
1 cup Sugar
½ cup Olive oil
4 drops Lavender essential oil
Dried Lavender (optional)

Directions:
In a large bowl, add sugar. Mix in olive oil and combine thoroughly. Add lavender essential oil drop by drop, until scent strength is achieved. For added color, add a small handful of dried lavender (optional).

Follow the general directions on how to use bath scrubs.

MINTY BATH SCRUB

Nothing perks your day up like the scent of fresh mint. Wintergreen oil has that clean woody mint-scent that sharpens the mind and lifts your spirits. For extra exfoliating effects, dried mint is added to this delightful bath scrub. Because wintergreen is known to have an aspirin-like effect, the oil may help alleviate pain and soreness.

Ingredients:
1 cup Sea salt
1/4 cup Apricot Kernel oil
1tsp dried mint of your choosing
2 drops Wintergreen essential oil*

Directions:
In a large bowl, combine first three ingredients. Add Wintergreen essential oil, drop by drop, until desired scent strength is achieved.

Follow the general directions on how to use bath scrubs.

*Wintergreen is not recommended for anyone who is a regular user of aspirin, is allergic to aspirin, or if you are taking coagulants. Keep out of the reach of children as wintergreen oil may be harmful if swallowed. Call the poison control center or emergency room right away if the oil is consumed.

LEMON BATH SCRUB

The refreshing scent of lemon comes alive in the bath or shower and helps remove dry skin in this bracing scrub.

Ingredients:
1 cup Sea salt
1/4 cup Sweet Almond oil
1tsp lemon zest
2 drops lemon essential oil

Directions:
In a large bowl, combine first three ingredients well. Add lemon essential oil drop by drop until desired scent strength is achieved.

Follow the general directions on how to use bath scrubs.

Conclusion

We've come to the end of this Art of the Bath collection of bath recipes. If you're like me, you can't wait to have them on hand and ready to use whenever you want some in-home spa time. Whatever your mood, there's a bomb, melt, scrub, or salt recipe ready and waiting.

Don't forget that these bath products are also unique, handmade gifts. Not only can these recipes provide *you* with bath salts, scrubs, bath bombs, and melts and turn your next bath into a luxurious spa moment, they can do the same thing for family and friends. Why not share the healing, meditative, and spiritually renewing benefits these bath aids provide with others?

Be sure and look for my other books that relate to the whole "art of the bath" experience and tell others.

Alynda Carroll

PS: I hope you've enjoyed this book and will take a few minutes to leave a review. Reviews are a big help for authors as well as readers.

About the Author

Alynda Carroll has loved baths since she was a little girl. Bubble baths, lotions, and creams have fascinated her. She spent many hours watching her mom create homemade beauty recipes. Later, Alynda's interests expanded to include herbs, essential oils, aromatherapy and the art of the bath as it is today.

Be sure and buy the rest of Alynda Carroll's best-selling books that make up her popular series The Art of the Bath, s well as her new series Life Hacks for Everyday Living. Look for the excerpt from her new book HOUSEHOLD HACKS at the back of this book.

MORE BOOKS BY ALYNDA CARROLL

The Art of the Bath Series

Custom Massage Therapy Oils: A DIY Guide to Therapeutic Recipes for Homemade Massage Oils

A DIY Guide to Therapeutic Bath Enhancements: Homemade Recipes for Bath Salts, Melts, Bombs & Scrubs

A DIY Guide to Therapeutic Body & Skin Care Recipes: Homemade Body Lotions, Skin Creams, Gels, Whipped Butters, Herbal Balms & Salves

A DIY Guide to Therapeutic Spa Treatments: Homemade Recipes for the Face, Hands, Feet & Body

A DIY Guide to Therapeutic Body Butters: A Beginner's Guide to Homemade Body and Hair Butters

A DIY Guide to Therapeutic Natural Hair Care Recipes: A Beginner's Guide to Homemade Shampoos, Conditioners, Rinses, Gels and Sprays

Life Hacks for Everyday Living *(New Series)*

HOUSEHOLD HACKS: Super Simple Ways to Clean Your Home Effortlessly Using Hydrogen Peroxide and Other Cleaning Secrets

What's New?

Turn the page to read an excerpt from HOUSEHOLD HACKS. To receive updates on the release of Alynda Carroll's next books in the Art of the Bath series and BEAUTY HACKS, go to:

www.SimpleLivingHacks.com

Excerpt from
HOUSEHOLD HACKS

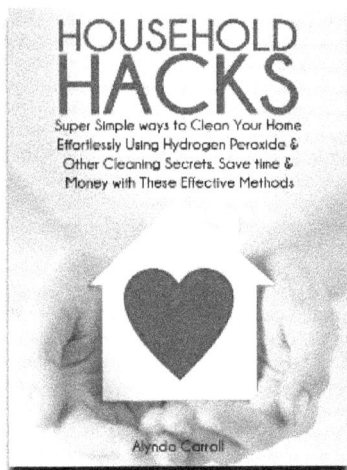

Welcome to Household Hacks, my personal collection of more than 200 cleaning tips, tricks, and household hacks for all areas of the home with an emphasis on using natural, inexpensive cleaners and strategies. Many have been around for a long time, but others are focused on the way we live today.

The advantages are many. You'll save money, time, and energy. You'll also become more effective at housecleaning by using these tips and strategies that will free up your time.

You'll find information about well-seasoned natural cleaners that have been helping people clean for generations and understand why they are gaining popularity today.

You'll discover cleaning strategies and hacks for various rooms including the kitchen, bathroom, and bedroom, as well as the home office. You'll even find creative living hacks to make home life easier.

This collection captures my favorites and includes additional hints and alternatives. If you already have a deep interest in DIY household hacks and natural cleaners, you will probably come across some familiar cleaning remedies. They will serve as reminders, but be of more interest to readers who are just starting down this more natural and simplified way of living. However, newer strategies and ideas will encourage you on your own journey toward living a more natural, clean, and simple life.

A major plus about having this book is that everything is gathered in this one place. This is a good, fun, and definitely useful reference to have on hand.

How the Book is Organized

The book begins by taking a look at the top natural cleaners in use today. There are several cleaning hacks and tips for each cleaner. I like to have a list of things I can do with a particular cleaner, as well a collection of cleaning tips particular to an area of the home. The second section offers additional cleaning suggestions and creative household hacks for the kitchen, bathroom, bedroom, laundry and closet, living room, home office, and, by extension, the car.

- ❑ Natural Cleaners
- ❑ Hydrogen Peroxide
- ❑ Vinegar
- ❑ Baking Soda
- ❑ Lemon and lemon juice
- ❑ Apple Cider Vinegar
- ❑ Salt
- ❑ Household Hacks
- ❑ Office and Technology
- ❑ Bathroom
- ❑ Kitchen
- ❑ Bedroom
- ❑ Laundry and Closet
- ❑ Car
- ❑ Creative Hacks

Now that you have an idea of what *HOUSEHOLD HACKS* contains, are you ready to discover its treasures?

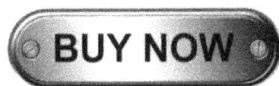

BUY NOW

Buy your copy of *HOUSEHOLD HACKS* today.
www.SimpleLivingHacks.com

NOTES

INDEX

www.ingramcontent.com/pod-product-compliance
Lightning Source LLC
Chambersburg PA
CBHW022125280326
41933CB00007B/553